The Ultimate Slow Cooker Breakfast Cookbook

Quick and Easy Tasty Recipes To Start Your Day Affordable For Beginners

Laurel Twitty

advice. The content within this book has been derived from various sources. Please consult a licensed professional before attempting any techniques outlined in this book.

By reading this document, the reader agrees that under no circumstances is the author responsible for any losses, direct or indirect, which are incurred as a result of the use of information contained within this document, including, but not limited to, — errors, omissions, or inaccuracies.

Table of contents

Cinnamon Raisin Steel-Cut Oatmeal

Preparation time: 5 minutes

Cooking time: 8 hours

Servings: 2

Ingredients:

- ¾ cup steel-cut oats
- ¼ cup raisins
- 1 teaspoon ground cinnamon
- 1/8 teaspoon sea salt
- 3 cups almond milk or water

Directions:

1. Put the oats, raisins, cinnamon, and salt in the slow cooker and stir to combine. Pour in the almond milk and stir.
2. Put cover and cook the oatmeal on low for 8 hours or overnight.

Nutrition: Calories: 293 Saturated Fat: 1g Trans Fat: 0g
Carbohydrates: 56g Fiber: 7g Sodium: 132mg Protein: 10g

Pear Chai-Spiced Oatmeal

Preparation time: 5 minutes

Cooking time: 8 hours

Servings: 4

Ingredients:

- ¾ cup steel-cut oats
- 1/8 teaspoon ground cardamom
- 1/8 teaspoon ground nutmeg
- 1/8 teaspoon ground ginger
- ¼ teaspoon cinnamon
- 1/8 teaspoon sea salt
- 1 ripe pear, cored, peeled, and diced
- 3 cups unsweetened almond milk or water

Directions:

1. Put the oats, cardamom, nutmeg, ginger, cinnamon, and salt in the slow cooker and stir to combine. Stir in the pear and the almond milk.
2. Put cover and cook the oatmeal on low for 8 hours or overnight.

Nutrition: Calories: 324 Saturated Fat: 1g Trans Fat: 0g Carbohydrates: 53g Fiber: 10g Sodium: 343mg Protein: 11g

Pumpkin Spice Oatmeal

Preparation time: 5 minutes

Cooking time: 6 hours

Servings: 4

Ingredients:

- ¾ cup steel-cut oats
- 1 teaspoon ground cinnamon
- 1/8 teaspoon ground ginger
- 1/8 teaspoon ground nutmeg
- 1/8 teaspoon ground cloves
- 1/8 teaspoon sea salt
- 1 cup pumpkin purée
- 2 cups unsweetened almond milk or water

Directions:

1. Mix the oats, cinnamon, ginger, nutmeg, cloves, and salt in the slow cooker.
2. whisk together the pumpkin and almond milk and pour the mixture into the oats in bowl.
3. Stir gently to combine the ingredients.
4. Put cover and cook the oatmeal on low for 8 hours or overnight.

Nutrition: Calories: 313 Saturated Fat: 2g Trans Fat: 0g Carbohydrates: 54g Fiber: 15g Sodium: 275mg Protein: 13g

Breakfast Quinoa & Fruit

Preparation time: 5minutes

Cooking time: 6 hours

Servings: 4

Ingredients:

- ¾ cup quinoa
- 2 cups fresh fruit
- 1/8 teaspoon sea salt
- 1 teaspoon vanilla extract
- 3 cups water
- 2 tablespoons toasted pecans, for garnish

Directions:

1. Place the fruit, quinoa and salt in the slow cooker.
2. Add in the vanilla extract and water, and mix
3. Put cover and cook on low for 8 hours or overnight.
4. Garnish each serving with a sprinkle of the toasted pecans.

Nutrition: Calories: 311 Saturated Fat: 1g Trans Fat: 0g Carbohydrates: 52g Fiber: 13g Sodium: 273mg Protein: 12g

Strawberry Cream Cheese French Toast

Preparation time: 10 minutes

Cooking time: 6 hours

Servings: 2

Ingredients:

- 1 teaspoon butter, at room temperature
- 2 eggs
- ½ cup 2% milk
- 1 teaspoon vanilla extract
- 1/8 teaspoon sea salt
- 5 slices whole-grain bread
- 2 cups fresh strawberries
- 2 ounces' low-fat cream cheese, cut into small chunks

Directions:

1. Oil the inside of the slow cooker with the butter.
2. whisk together the eggs, milk, vanilla, and salt in a large bowl.
3. Toss the bread cubes in this mixture until they are thoroughly saturated.
4. Pour half of the bread mixture into the slow cooker.
5. Top with the strawberries and cream cheese. Add the remaining bread mixture.

6. Cover and cook on low for 6 hours or on high for 2½
    hours. To prepare the dish the night before, set a
    timer to turn on the slow cooker (set on low) one
    hour after you go to bed and turn off one hour
    before you plan to eat breakfast, for a total cook
    time of 6 hours.

Nutrition: Calories: 391 Saturated Fat: 10g Trans Fat: 0g
Carbohydrates: 40g Fiber: 7g Sodium: 606mg Protein: 17g

Cherry-Studded Quinoa Porridge

Preparation time: 5minutes

Cooking time: 6 hours

Servings: 4

Ingredients:

- ¾ cup quinoa
- ½ cup dried cherries
- 1/8 teaspoon sea salt
- 1 teaspoon vanilla extract
- 3 cups almond milk or water

Directions:

1. Place the quinoa, cherries, and salt in the slow cooker.
2. Pour in the vanilla and almond milk, and mix all of the ingredients together.
3. Put cover and cook on low for 8 hours or overnight.

Nutrition: Calories: 426 Saturated Fat: 0g Trans Fat: 0g Carbohydrates: 78g Fiber: 16g Sodium: 352mg Protein: 12g

Banana Nut French Toast

Preparation time: 10 minutes

Cooking time: 6 hours

Servings: 2

Ingredients:

- 2 eggs
- ¾ cup 2% milk
- 1 teaspoon vanilla extract
- 1 teaspoon ground cinnamon
- ¼ teaspoon ground nutmeg
- 1/8 teaspoon sea salt
- 2 cups sliced bananas
- 5 slices whole-grain bread
- 1 tablespoon finely chopped toasted pecans

Directions:

1. Oil the inside of the slow cooker with the butter.
2. whisk together the eggs, milk, vanilla, cinnamon, nutmeg, and salt. Gently toss the bananas and bread cubes in the mixture until the bread is thoroughly saturated.
3. Pour the bread and banana mixture into the slow cooker. Sprinkle the top with the toasted pecans.
4. Put cover and cook on low for 4 hours or on high for 2 hours.

Nutrition: Calories: 423 Saturated Fat: 5g Trans Fat: 0g
Carbohydrates: 59g Fiber: 9gSodium: 537mg Protein: 17g

Yogurt with Mangos & Cardamom

Preparation time: 10 minutes

Cooking time: 6 hours

Servings: 4

Ingredients:

- 4 cups 2% milk
- ¼ cup plain yogurt with live cultures
- 2 mangos, cut into chunks
- 1 tablespoon honey
- ¼ teaspoon ground cardamom

Directions:

1. Transfer the milk into the slow cooker. Put cover and cook on low for 1 hours.

2. Unplug the slow cooker and stir in the yogurt. Cover with the lid and wrap the outside of the slow cooker housing with a bath towel to help insulate it. Allow it to rest for 8 hours or overnight.

3. For a thick yogurt, strain the mixture in a medium bowl through a few cheesecloth layers for 12 to 15 minutes.

Nutrition: Calories: 206 Saturated Fat: 3g Trans Fat: 0g Carbohydrates: 31g Fiber: 2g Sodium: 128mg Protein: 9g

Yogurt & Berry Parfait

Preparation time: 10 minutes

Cooking time: 6 hours

Servings: 4

Ingredients:

- 4 cups 2% milk
- ¼ cup plain yogurt with live cultures
- 2 cups blueberries
- 1 cup low-fat, low-sugar granola

Directions:

1. Transfer the milk into the slow cooker. Cover and cook on low for 1 hours.
2. Unplug the slow cooker and stir in the yogurt. Put the lid on and wrap the slow cooker in a bath towel to help insulate it. Allow the yogurt to rest for 8 hours or overnight.
3. strain the mixture into a medium bowl through a few cheesecloth layers for 11 to 15 minutes for the thick yogurt
4. layer the strained yogurt with the berries and the granola.

Nutrition: Calories: 266 Saturated Fat: 4g Trans Fat: 0g Carbohydrates: 44g Fiber: 4g Sodium: 183mg Protein: 11g

Southwest Sweet Potato & Corn Scramble

Preparation time: 10 minutes

Cooking time: 6 hours

Servings: 2

Ingredients:

- 1 teaspoon butter, at room temperature, or extra-virgin olive oil
- 4 eggs
- ½ cup 2% milk
- 1/8 teaspoon sea salt
- ½ teaspoon smoked paprika
- ½ teaspoon ground cumin
- Freshly ground black pepper
- 1 cup finely diced sweet potato
- 1 cup frozen corn kernels, thawed
- ½ cup diced roasted red peppers
- 2 tablespoons minced onion

Directions:

1. Oil the inside of the slow cooker with the butter.
2. In small bowl, whisk together the eggs, milk, salt, paprika, and cumin. Season with the freshly ground black pepper.

3. Put the sweet potato, corn, red pepper, and onion
    into the slow cooker. Pour in the egg mixture and
    stir gently.

4. Put cover and cook on low for 8 hours or overnight.

Nutrition: Calories: 349 Saturated Fat: 5g Trans Fat: 0g
Carbohydrates: 45g Fiber: 6g Sodium: 430mg Protein: 18g

Smoked Salmon & Potato Casserole

Preparation time: 10 minutes

Cooking time: 6 hours

Servings: 2

Ingredients:

- 1 teaspoon butter, at room temperature, or extra-virgin olive oil
- 2 eggs
- 1 cup 2% milk
- 1 teaspoon dried dill
- 1/8 teaspoon sea salt
- Freshly ground black pepper
- 2 medium russet potatoes
- 4 ounces smoked salmon

Directions:

1. Oil the inside of the slow cooker with the butter.
2. whisk together the eggs, milk, dill, salt, and a few black pepper grinds in a bowl.
3. Spread one-third of the potatoes in a single layer on the bottom of the slow cooker and top them with one-third of the salmon. Transfer one-third of the egg mixture over the salmon. Repeat this layering with the remaining potatoes, salmon, and egg mixture.
4. Put cover and cook on low for 8 hours or overnight.

Nutrition: Calories: 355 Saturated Fat: 5g Trans Fat: 0g

Carbohydrates: 40g Fiber: 5g Sodium: 1397mg Protein: 24g

Prosciutto, Rosemary & Potato Breakfast Casserole

Preparation time: 10 minutes

Cooking time: 6 hours

Servings: 2

Ingredients:

- 1 teaspoon butter, at room temperature, or extra-virgin olive oil
- 4 eggs
- ½ cup 2% milk
- 1 tablespoon minced fresh rosemary
- 1/8 teaspoon sea salt
- Freshly ground black pepper
- 2 medium russet potatoes, peeled and sliced thin
- 2 ounces' prosciutto

Directions:

1. Oil the inside of the slow cooker with the butter.
2. whisk together the eggs, milk, rosemary, salt, and a few black pepper grinds in a small bowl.
3. Layer one-third of the potatoes in lowest of the slow cooker and top that layer with one-third of the prosciutto. Transfer one-third of the egg mixture over the prosciutto. Repeat this layering with the remaining ingredients.
4. Put cover and cook on low for 8 hours or overnight.

Nutrition: Calories: 367 Saturated Fat: 5g Trans Fat: 0g
Carbohydrates: 39g Fiber: 6g Sodium: 637mg Protein: 23g

Ham & Cheese Breakfast Casserole

Preparation time: 10 minutes

Cooking time: 6 hours

Servings: 2

Ingredients:

- 1 teaspoon butter, at room temperature, or extra-virgin olive oil
- 2 eggs
- 2 egg whites
- Freshly ground black pepper
- 2 slices whole-grain bread, crusts removed, cut into 1-inch cubes
- 2 ounces aged ham, diced
- 2 ounces' hard cheese, such as Parmesan, shredded

Directions:

1. Oil the inside of the slow cooker with the butter.
2. whisk together the eggs, egg whites, and a few black pepper grinds in a small bowl.
3. Put the bread, ham, and cheese in the slow cooker. Transfer the egg mixture over the top and stir gently to combine.
4. Put cover and cook on low for 8 hours or overnight.

Nutrition: Calories: 324 Saturated Fat: 8g Trans Fat: 0g Carbohydrates: 19g Fiber: 5g Sodium: 866mg Protein: 27g

Southwest Breakfast Casserole

Preparation time: 10 minutes

Cooking time: 6 hours

Servings: 2

Ingredients:

- 1 teaspoon butter, at room temperature, or extra-virgin olive oil
- 2 eggs
- 2 egg whites
- 1 teaspoon ground cumin
- 1 teaspoon smoked paprika
- 1/8 teaspoon sea salt
- Freshly ground black pepper
- ½ cup shredded pepper Jack cheese
- ½ cup canned fire-roasted diced tomatoes
- ½ cup canned black beans, drained and rinsed
- 1 teaspoon minced garlic
- 3 corn tortillas
- ¼ cup fresh cilantro, for garnish

Directions:

1. Oil the inside of the slow cooker with the butter.
2. In a small bowl, whisk together the eggs, egg whites, cumin, paprika, salt, and a few black pepper grinds.

3. In a separate small bowl, combine the cheese, tomatoes, black beans, and garlic.

4. Place one of the corn tortillas in the slow cooker and top it with half of the cheese and bean mixture. Transfer one-third of the egg mixture over the top of the cheese and beans. Top the egg mixture with another tortilla. Top that tortilla with the remaining cheese and bean mixture, followed by one-third of the egg mixture. Place the last tortilla on top of the egg mixture, and then pour the remaining egg mixture over the top of it.

5. Put cover and cook on low for 8 hours or overnight. Garnish with the fresh cilantro before serving.

Nutrition: Calories: 366 Saturated Fat: 9g Trans Fat: 0g Carbohydrates: 31g Fiber: 8g Sodium: 640mg Protein: 24g

Zucchini-Carrot Bread

Preparation Time: 15 Minutes

Cooking Time: 3 or 5 Hours

Servings: 8

Ingredients:

- 2 teaspoons butter, for greasing pan
- 1 cup almond flour
- 1 cup granulated erythritol
- ½ cup coconut flour
- 1½ teaspoons baking powder
- 1 teaspoon ground cinnamon
- ½ teaspoon ground nutmeg
- ½ teaspoon baking soda
- ¼ teaspoon salt
- 4 eggs
- ½ cup butter, melted
- 1 tablespoon pure vanilla extract
- 1½ cups finely grated zucchini
- ½ cup finely grated carrot

Directions:

1. Lightly grease a 9-by-5-inch loaf pan with the butter and set aside.

2. Place a small rack in the bottom of your slow cooker.

3. In a large bowl, stir together the almond flour, erythritol, coconut flour, baking powder, cinnamon, nutmeg, baking soda, and salt until well mixed.

4. In a separate medium bowl, whisk together the eggs, melted butter, and vanilla until well blended.

5. Add the wet fixings to dry fixings and stir to combine.

6. Stir in the zucchini and carrot.

7. Spoon the batter into the prepared loaf pan.

8. Place the loaf pan on the rack in the bottom of the slow cooker, cover, and cook on high for 3 hours.

9. Remove the loaf pan, let the bread cool completely, and serve.

Nutrition: Calories: 217 Total Fat: 19g Protein: 8g Total Carbs: 5g Fiber: 3g Net Carbs: 2g Cholesterol: 136mg

Keto Granola

Preparation Time: 10 Minutes

Cooking Time: 3 to 4 Hours

Servings: 16

Ingredients:

- ½ Cup coconut oil, melted
- 2 teaspoons pure vanilla extract
- 1 teaspoon maple extract
- 1 cup chopped pecans
- 1 cup sunflower seeds
- 1 cup unsweetened shredded coconut
- ½ cup hazelnuts
- ½ cup slivered almonds
- ¼ cup granulated erythritol
- ½ teaspoon cinnamon
- ¼ teaspoon ground nutmeg
- ¼ teaspoon salt

Directions:

1. Grease the slow cooker with 1 tablespoon of the coconut oil.

2. In a large bowl, whisk together the remaining coconut oil, vanilla, and maple extract. Add the pecans, sunflower seeds, coconut, hazelnuts,

almonds, erythritol, cinnamon, nutmeg, and salt. Toss to coat the nuts and seeds.

3.   Transfer the mixture to the insert.

4.   Cover then cook on low for 3 to 4 hours, until the granola is crispy.

5.   Transfer the granola to a baking sheet covered in parchment or foil to cool.

6.   Store in a sealed container in the refrigerator for up to 2 weeks.

Nutrition: Calories: 236 Total Fat: 23g Protein: 6g Total Carbs: 5g Fiber: 3g Net Carbs: 2g Cholesterol: 0mg

Pumpkin-Pie Breakfast Bars

Preparation Time: 15 Minutes

Cooking Time: 3 Hours

Servings: 8

Ingredients:

For the crust

- 5 tablespoons butter, softened, divided
- ¾ cup unsweetened shredded coconut
- ½ cup almond flour
- ¼ cup granulated erythritol
- For the filling
- 1 (28-ounce) can pumpkin purée
- 1 cup heavy (whipping) cream
- 4 eggs
- 1-ounce protein powder
- 1 teaspoon pure vanilla extract
- 4 drops liquid stevia
- 1 teaspoon ground cinnamon
- ½ teaspoon ground ginger
- ¼ teaspoon ground nutmeg
- Pinch ground cloves
- Pinch salt

Directions:

1. For the crust

2. Lightly grease the bottom of the insert of the slow cooker with 1 tablespoon of the butter.

3. In a small bowl, stir together the coconut, almond flour, erythritol, and remaining butter until the mixture forms into coarse crumbs.

4. Press the crumbs into the bottom of the insert evenly to form a crust.

5. For the filling

6. In a medium bowl, stir the pumpkin, heavy cream, eggs, protein powder, vanilla, stevia, cinnamon, ginger, nutmeg, cloves, and salt until well blended.

7. Spread the filling evenly over the crust.

8. Cover and cook on low for 3 hours.

9. Uncover and let cool for 30 minutes. Then place the insert in the refrigerator until completely chilled, about 2 hours.

10. Slice into squares and store them in the refrigerator in a sealed container for up to 5 days.

Nutrition: Calories: 227 Total Fat: 19g Protein: 10g Total Carbs: 8g Fiber: 4g Net Carbs: 4g Cholesterol: 143mg

Nutty "Oatmeal"

Preparation Time: 10 Minutes

Cooking Time: 8 Hours

Servings: 6

Ingredients:

- 1 tablespoon coconut oil
- 1 cup coconut milk
- 1 cup unsweetened shredded coconut
- ½ cup chopped pecans
- ½ cup sliced almonds
- ¼ cup granulated erythritol
- 1 avocado, diced
- 2 ounces protein powder
- 1 teaspoon ground cinnamon
- ¼ teaspoon ground nutmeg
- ½ cup blueberries, for garnish

Directions:

1. Lightly grease the insert of a slower cooker with the coconut oil.

2. Place the coconut milk, shredded coconut, pecans, almonds, erythritol, avocado, protein powder, cinnamon, and nutmeg in the slow cooker.

3. Cover then cook on low for 8 hours.

4. Stir the mixture to create the desired texture.

5. Serve topped with the blueberries.

Nutrition: Calories: 365 Total Fat: 33g Protein: 14g Total Carbs: 10g Fiber: 6g Net Carbs: 4g Cholesterol: 0mg

Pumpkin-Pecan N' Oatmeal

Preparation Time: 10 Minutes

Cooking Time: 8 Hours

Servings: 4

Ingredients:

- 1 tablespoon coconut oil
- 3 cups cubed pumpkin, cut into 1-inch chunks
- 2 cups coconut milk
- ½ cup ground pecans
- 1-ounce plain protein powder
- 2 tablespoons granulated erythritol
- 1 teaspoon maple extract
- ½ teaspoon ground nutmeg
- ¼ teaspoon ground cinnamon
- Pinch ground allspice

Directions:

1. Lightly grease the insert of a slower cooker with the coconut oil.

2. Place the pumpkin, coconut milk, pecans, protein powder, erythritol, maple extract, nutmeg, cinnamon, and allspice in the insert.

3. Cover then cook on low for 8 hours.

4. Stir the mixture or use a potato masher to create your preferred texture, and serve.

Nutrition: Calories: 292 Total Fat: 26g Protein: 10g Total Carbs: 9g Fiber: 2gNet Carbs: 7g Cholesterol: 0mg

Pumpkin-Nutmeg Pudding

Preparation Time: 15 Minutes

Cooking Time: 6 to 7 Hours

Servings: 8

Ingredients:

- ¼ Cup melted butter, divided
- 2½ cups canned pumpkin purée
- 2 cups coconut milk
- 4 eggs
- 1 tablespoon pure vanilla extract
- 1 cup almond flour
- ½ cup granulated erythritol
- 2 ounces protein powder
- 1 teaspoon baking powder
- 1 teaspoon ground cinnamon
- ¼ teaspoon ground nutmeg
- Pinch ground cloves

Directions:

1. Grease the insert of the slow cooker with 1 tablespoon of the butter.

2. In a large bowl, whisk together the remaining butter, pumpkin, coconut milk, eggs, and vanilla until well blended.

3. In a small bowl, stir together the almond flour, erythritol, protein powder, baking powder, cinnamon, nutmeg, and cloves.

4. Add the dry fixings to the wet fixings and stir to combine.

5. Pour the mixture into the insert.

6. Cover then cook on low for 6 to 7 hours.

7. Serve warm.

Nutrition: Calories: 265 Total Fat: 22g Protein: 13g Total Carbs: 8g Fiber: 3g Net Carbs: 5g Cholesterol: 121mg

Scrambled Eggs with Smoked Salmon

Preparation time: 15 minutes

Cooking time: 2 hours

Servings: 6

Ingredients:

- Smoked salmon ¼ lb.
- eggs12 pcs fresh
- heavy cream½ cup
- almond flour¼ cup
- Salt and black pepper at will
- Butter2 tablespoons
- fresh chives at will

Directions:

1. Cut the slices of salmon. Set aside for garnish. Chop the rest of the salmon into small pieces.
2. Take a medium bowl, whisk the eggs and cream together. Add half of the chopped chives, season eggs with salt and pepper. Add flour.
3. Dissolve the butter over medium heat, then pour into the mixture. Grease the Slow Cooker with oil or cooking spray.
4. Add salmon pieces to the mixture, pour it into the Slow Cooker. Set to cook on low within 2 hours.
5. Garnish the dish with remaining salmon, chives. Serve warm and enjoy!

Nutrition: Calories: 263 Carbs: 0g Fat: 0g Protein: 0g

Garlic-Parmesan Asparagus Crock Pot

Preparation time: 15 minutes

Cooking time: 1 hour

Servings: 6

Ingredients:

- olive oil extra virgin2 tablespoons
- minced garlic2 teaspoons
- egg 1 pcs fresh
- garlic salt1/2 teaspoon
- fresh asparagus12 ounces
- Parmesan cheese1/3 cup
- Pepper at will

Directions:

1. Peel the garlic and mince it. Wash the asparagus. Shred the Parmesan cheese.
2. Take a medium-sized bowl combine oil, garlic, cracked egg, and salt together. Whisk everything well.
3. Cover the green beans and coat them well.
4. Spread the cooking spray over the Slow Cooker's bottom, put the coated asparagus, season with the shredded cheese. Toss.
5. Cook on high within 1 hour. Once the time is over, you may also season with the rest of the cheese. Serve.

42

Persian Omelet Crock Pot

Preparation time: 15 minutes

Cooking time: 3 hours

Servings: 14

Ingredients:

- olive oil 2 tablespoons
- butter 1 tablespoons
- red onion 1 large
- green onions 4 pcs
- garlic 2 cloves
- Spinach 2 oz.
- fresh chives ¼ cup
- cilantro leaves ¼ cup
- parsley leaves ¼ cup
- fresh dill 2 tablespoons
- Kosher salt and black pepper at will
- pine nuts ¼ cup
- eggs 9 large
- whole milk ¼ cup
- Greek yogurt 1 cup

Directions:

1. Take a saucepan to melt the butter. Add red onion, stirring occasionally; it takes about 8-9 minutes.
2. Add green onions, garlic, continue cooking for 4 minutes. Put the spinach, chives, parsley, and

cilantro, add salt and pepper at will. Remove the skillet, add the pine nuts.

3. Take a bowl, crack the eggs, add milk, and a little pepper and whisk. Mix the eggs with veggie mixture.

4. Open the Slow Cooker and spread the cooking spray over the bottom and sides. Pour the mix into the Slow Cooker. Cook on low for 3 hours. Serve with Greek yogurt. Bon Appetite!

Nutrition: Calories: 220 Carbs: 9g Fat: 16g Protein: 12g

Broccoli and Cheese Stuffed Squash

Preparation time: 15 minutes

Cooking time: 3 hours

Servings: 7

Ingredients:

- squash 1 pcs, halves
- broccoli florets 2 cups
- garlic 3 pcs
- red pepper flakes 1 teaspoon
- Italian season 1 teaspoon
- mozzarella cheese 1/2 cup
- Parmesan cheese 1/3 cup
- cooking spray
- salt and pepper at will

Directions:

1. Grease the Slow Cooker. Put the squash halves in the Slow Cooker.
2. Add a little bit of water at room temperature to the bottom of the Slow Cooker.
3. Put on low within 2 hours, until squash is mild. Take off the squash and let it cool for about 15 minutes.
4. Take a medium skillet, add pepper flakes and a little bit oil and cook for 20 seconds, stir it continuously.
5. Add broccoli, minced garlic to the skillet, continue to stir thoroughly, until the broccoli is tender.

6. Take the squash and using a fork; take off the flesh of the squash. Add it to the medium bowl and conjoin with the broccoli mixture.

7. Shred the Parmesan cheese carefully, put salt and pepper at will, and add seasoning to the mixture. Mix well and fill the squash.

8. Put the filled squash again in the Slow Cooker, dress with mozzarella cheese each squash half.

9. Cover and cook on low within 1 hour. Remove the dish and serve.

Nutrition: Calories: 230 Carbs: 22g Fat: 6g Protein: 21g

Garlic Butter Keto Spinach

Preparation time: 15 minutes

Cooking time: 1 hour

Servings: 4

Ingredients:

- salted butter 2 tablespoons
- garlic, minced 4 cloves
- Baby spinach 8 oz.
- Pinch of salt
- lemon juice 1 teaspoons

Directions:

1. Heat-up a little skillet, add the butter, and melt. Sautee the garlic until a bit tender.
2. Spray the cooking spray over the bottom of the Slow Cooker.
3. Put the spinach into the Slow Cooker, season with salt and lemon juice, tender garlic, butter.
4. Put to cook on low within 1 hour. Garnish with fresh lemon wedges. Serve hot.

Nutrition: Calories: 38 Carbs: 2g Fat: 3g Protein: 2g

Keto Crock Pot Tasty Onions

Preparation time: 15 minutes

Cooking time: 6 hours

Servings: 4

Ingredients:

- Onions 4 (or 5) large pcs, sliced
- Butter or coconut oil 4 tablespoon
- Coconut aminos 1/4 cup
- Splenda (optional)
- Salt and pepper

Directions:

1. Place the onion slices into the Slow Cooker. Top the onion slices with coconut amino and butter; you might add Splenda at will.
2. Cook it on low during 6-7 hours. Serve over the grilled vegetables.

Nutrition: Calories: 38 Carbs: 9g Fat: 0g Protein: 0g

Crock Pot Benedict Casserole

Preparation time: 15 minutes

Cooking time: 4 hours

Servings: 7

Ingredients:

- For the Casserole
- English muffin 1 large, cut into portions
- Canadian bacon1 lb. thick-cut
- eggs 10 large
- milk 1 cup
- salt and pepper
- for garnish
- For the Sauce
- egg 6 yolks
- lemon juice 1 1/2 tablespoon
- unsalted butter, melted1 1/2 sticks
- salt
- pinch of cayenne

Directions:

1. For the muffin: Using a medium-sized skillet, melt the butter. Add coconut and almond flour, egg, salt, and stir everything well. Add baking soda. Grease the Slow Cooker with cooking spray. Pour the mixture, put on low for 2 hours. Remove once done.

2. Grease again the Slow Cooker with cooking spray, cut the muffin into equal pieces, put on the bottom.
3. Slice the bacon, sprinkle half of it over top of the muffin pieces.
4. Whisk milk, eggs, season with salt and black pepper in a large bowl.
5. Pour the egg batter evenly over the muffin pieces and top with the rest of the bacon.
6. Cook on low within 2 hours in the slow cooker. Remove, and keep the muffins covered before serving.
7. To make the sauce, set up a double boiler, put the egg yolks, squeeze lemon juice in a bowl, and mix.
8. Put your bowl over the double boiler, continue whisking carefully; the bowl mustn't get too hot.
9. Put in the melted butter while continuing to whisk.
10. Season with salt and pepper. You may also add a little bit more lemon juice or cayenne.
11. Serve and enjoy.

Nutrition: Calories: 286 Carbs: 16g Fat: 19g Protein: 14g

Crustless Crock Pot Spinach Quiche

Preparation time: 15 minutes

Cooking time: 2 hours

Servings: 11

Ingredients:

- Frozen spinach10 oz. package
- Butter or ghee1 tablespoon
- Red bell pepper1 medium
- Cheddar cheese1 1/2 cups
- Eggs8 pcs
- Homemade sour cream1 cup
- Fresh chives2 tablespoons
- Sea salt1/2 teaspoon
- Ground black pepper1/4 teaspoon
- Ground almond flour   1/2 cup
- Baking soda1/4 teaspoon

Directions:

1. Let the frozen spinach thaw and drain it well. Chop finely. Wash the pepper and slice it. Remove the seeds.
2. Grate the cheddar cheese and set aside. Chop the fresh chives finely.
3. Grease the slow cooker with cooking spray.
4. Take a little skillet, heat the butter over high heat on the stove, sauté the pepper until tender, for

about 6 minutes. Mix the eggs, sour cream, salt, plus pepper in a large bowl.

5. Add grated cheese and chives and continue to mix. In another medium-sized bowl, combine almond flour with baking soda.

6. Pour into the egg mixture, add peppers to the egg's mixture, and pour gently into the slow cooker.

7. Set to cook on high within 2 hours then Serve.

Nutrition: Calories: 153 Carbs: 19g Fat: 3g Protein: 9g

Broccoli Gratin with Parmesan and Swiss Cheese

Preparation time: 15 minutes

Cooking time: 1 hour

Servings: 7

Ingredients:

- bite-size broccoli flowerets8 cups
- Swiss cheese1 1/2 cups
- mayo 8 teaspoon
- lemon juice1 1/2 tablespoon
- Dijon mustard3/4 teaspoon
- green onions3 tablespoon
- Parmesan cheese1/4 cup
- black pepper and salt to taste

Directions:

1. Wash broccoli and cut into small florets. Grate both parmesan and Swiss cheese into a bowl. Set aside.
2. Squeeze juice of a lemon into a cup. Wash and chop the green onions.
3. Grease with cooking spray or olive oil (optional) over the bottom of the slow cooker.
4. Put broccoli florets in a single layer. Mix in a separate bowl lemon juice, mustard, mayo, black pepper, add to the mixture green onion and grated cheese.

5. Put the mixture over the broccoli, cover, and cook on low 1 hour. Serve hot.

Nutrition: Calories: 210 Carbs: 44g Fat: 2g Protein: 5g

Crock Pot Cream Cheese French Toast

Preparation time: 15 minutes

Cooking time: 2 hours

Servings: 9

Ingredients:

- cream cheese 1 (8-oz) package
- slivered almonds ¼ cup
- keto bread 1 loaf
- eggs 4 pcs
- almond extract 1 teaspoon
- sweetener 1 tablespoon
- milk 1 cup
- butter 2 tablespoon
- Cheddar cheese ½ cup
- Maple syrup, at will, for dressing

Directions:

1. Mix cream cheese with almonds in a large bowl. Slice the keto bread into 2-inch slices. Try to make a 1/2-inch slit (horizontal) at the bottom of every piece to make a pocket.
2. Fill all the slices with cream mixture. Set aside. In a little bowl, mix eggs, extract the sweetener in milk. Coat the keto slices into the mix.
3. Grease with cooking spray the slow cooker over the bottom and sides, then put the coated keto slices

on the slow cooker's base. Put on the top of each separate piece additional shredded cheese.

4. Cook on low for 2 hours. Serve hot.

Nutrition: Calories: 280 Carbs: 34g Fat: 8g Protein: 19g

Keto Crock Pot Turkey Stuffed Peppers

Preparation time: 15 minutes

Cooking time: 6 hours

Servings: 7

Ingredients:

- olive oil1 tablespoon
- Ground turkey1 lb.
- onion1 pcs
- garlic1 clove
- green bell peppers4 pcs
- tomato sauce/pasta sauce (low carb)24 oz. jar
- water1/2 cup

Directions:

1. Peel and cut the small onion, peel the garlic, and press or mince it.
2. Wash the bell peppers, cut off the tops and clean them accurately.
3. Take a medium bowl, put their ground turkey, cut onion, pressed or minced garlic, and add pasta sauce.
4. Separate the compound into four equal parts, place the mixtures into the prepared cleaned peppers.

5. Spread the olive oil over the slow cooker bottom, and sides put the peppers inside, and top them with sauce.
6. Add a little water into the slow cooker, cook on low for 6-7 hours.
7. Serve with remaining sauce and enjoy.

Nutrition: Calories: 245 Carbs: 26g Fat: 7g Protein: 19g

Cherry Tomatoes Thyme Asparagus Frittata

Preparation time: 15 minutes

Cooking time: 6 hours

Servings: 6

Ingredients:

- 2 tablespoons unsalted butter, ghee, or extra-virgin olive oil
- 12 large eggs
- ¼ cup heavy (whipping) cream
- 1 tablespoon minced fresh thyme
- ½ teaspoon kosher salt
- ¼ teaspoon freshly ground black pepper
- 1½ cups shredded sharp white Cheddar cheese, divided
- ½ cup grated Parmesan cheese
- 16 cherry tomatoes
- 16 asparagus spears

Directions:

1. Glaze the inside of the slow cooker with the butter.
2. In the slow cooker, beat the eggs, then whisk in the heavy cream, thyme, salt, and pepper.
3. Add ¾ cup of Cheddar cheese and the Parmesan cheese and stir to mix.

4. Sprinkle the remaining ¾ cup of Cheddar cheese over the top. Scatter the cherry tomatoes over the frittata.

5. Arrange the asparagus spears decoratively over the top. Cook within 6 hours on low or 3 hours on soaring. Serve.

Nutrition: Calories: 370 Fat: 29g Carbs: 4g Protein: 24g

Healthy Low Carb Walnut Zucchini Bread

Preparation time: 15 minutes

Cooking time: 3 hours & 10 minutes

Servings: 12

Ingredients:

- 3 eggs
- 1/2 cup walnuts, chopped
- 2 cups zucchini, shredded
- 2 tsp vanilla
- 1/2 cup pure all-purpose sweetener
- 1/3 cup coconut oil, softened
- 1/2 tsp baking soda
- 1 1/2 Tsp baking powder
- 2 tsp cinnamon
- 1/3 cup coconut flour
- 1 cup almond flour
- 1/2 Tsp salt

Directions:

1. Mix the almond flour, baking powder, cinnamon, baking soda, coconut flour, and salt in a bowl. Set aside.

2. Whisk eggs, vanilla, sweetener, and oil in another bowl.
3. Put dry batter to the wet and fold well. Add walnut and zucchini and fold well.
4. Pour batter into the silicone bread pan. Place the bread pan into the slow cooker on the rack.
5. Cook on high within 3 hours. Cut the bread loaf into the slices and serve.

Nutrition: Calories: 174 Fat: 15.4 g Carb: 5.8 g Protein: 5.3 g

Savory Creamy Breakfast Casserole

Preparation time: 15 minutes

Cooking time: 6 hours

Servings: 8

Ingredients:

- 1 tablespoon unsalted butter, Ghee
- 10 large eggs, beaten
- 1 cup heavy (whipping) cream
- 1½ cups shredded sharp Cheddar cheese, divided
- ½ cup grated Romano cheese
- ½ teaspoon kosher salt
- ¼ teaspoon freshly ground black pepper
- 8 ounces thick-cut ham, diced
- ¾ head broccoli, cut into small florets
- ½ onion, diced

Directions:

1. Grease the slow cooker with the butter.
2. Whisk the eggs, heavy cream, ½ cup of Cheddar cheese, the Romano cheese, salt, and pepper inside the slow cooker.
3. Stir in the ham, broccoli, and onion. Put the remaining 1 cup of Cheddar cheese over the top.
4. Cook within 6 hours on low or 3 hours on high. Serve hot.

Nutrition: Calories: 465 Fat: 36g Carbs: 7g Protein: 28g

Low-Carb Hash Brown Breakfast Casserole

Preparation time: 15 minutes

Cooking time: 6 hours

Servings: 6

Ingredients:

- 1 tablespoon unsalted butter, Ghee
- 12 large eggs
- ½ cup heavy cream
- 1 teaspoon kosher salt
- ½ teaspoon ground black pepper
- ½ teaspoon ground mustard
- 1 head cauliflower, shredded or minced
- 1 onion, diced
- 10 ounces cooked sausage links, sliced
- 2 cups shredded Cheddar cheese, divided

Directions:

1. Grease the slow cooker with the butter.
2. Beat the eggs, then whisk in heavy cream, 1 teaspoon of salt, ½ teaspoon of pepper, and the ground mustard in a large bowl.
3. Spread about one-third of the cauliflower in an even layer in the bottom of the cooker.
4. Layer one-third of the onions over the cauliflower, then one-third of the sausage, and top with ½ cup

of Cheddar cheese. Season with salt and pepper. Repeat twice.

5. Pour the egg batter evenly over the layered Ingredients, then sprinkle the remaining ½ cup Cheddar cheese on top—Cook within 6 hours on low. Serve hot.

Nutrition: Calories: 523 Fat: 40g Carbs: 7g Protein: 33g

Onion Broccoli Cream Cheese Quiche

Preparation time: 15 minutes

Cooking time: 2 hours & 25 minutes

Servings: 8

Ingredients:

- 9 eggs
- 2 cups cheese, shredded and divided
- 8 oz. cream cheese
- 1/4 Tsp onion powder
- 3 cups broccoli, cut into florets
- 1/4 Tsp pepper
- 3/4 Tsp salt

Directions:

1. Add broccoli into the boiling water and cook for 3 minutes. Drain well and set aside to cool.
2. Add eggs, cream cheese, onion powder, pepper, and salt in mixing bowl and beat until well combined.
3. Spray slow cooker from inside using cooking spray.
4. Add cooked broccoli into the slow cooker then sprinkle half cup cheese.
5. Pour egg mixture over broccoli and cheese mixture.
6. Cook on high within 2 hours and 15 minutes.

7. Once it is done, then sprinkle the remaining cheese and cover for 10 minutes or until cheese melted. Serve.

Nutrition: Calories 296 Fat 24.3 g Carb 3.9 g Protein 16.4 g

Delicious Thyme Sausage Squash

Preparation time: 15 minutes

Cooking time: 6 hours

Servings: 4

Ingredients:

- 2 tablespoons extra-virgin olive oil
- 14 ounces smoked chicken sausage, thinly sliced
- ¼ cup chicken broth
- 1 onion, halved and sliced
- ½ medium butternut squash, peeled, diced
- 1 small green bell pepper, strips
- ½ small red bell pepper, strips
- ½ small yellow bell pepper, strips
- 2 teaspoons snipped fresh thyme or ½ teaspoon dried thyme, crushed
- ½ teaspoon kosher salt
- ½ teaspoon freshly ground black pepper
- 1 cup shredded Swiss cheese

Directions:

1. Combine the olive oil, sausage, broth, onion, butternut squash, bell peppers, thyme, salt, and pepper in the slow cooker. Toss to mix. Cook within 6 hours on low.

2. Before serving, sprinkle the Swiss cheese over the top, cover, and cook for about 3 minutes more to melt the cheese.

Nutrition: Calories: 502 Fat: 38g Carbs: 12g Protein: 27g

Mexican Style Breakfast Casserole

Preparation time: 15 minutes

Cooking time: 5 hours

Servings: 5

Ingredients:

- 5 eggs
- 6 ounces' pork sausage, cooked, drained
- ½ cup 1% milk
- ½ teaspoon garlic powder
- 2 jalapeños, deseeded, finely chopped
- ½ teaspoon ground cumin
- ½ teaspoon ground coriander
- 1 ½ cups chunky salsa
- 1 ½ cup pepper Jack cheese, shredded
- Salt to taste
- Pepper to taste
- ¼ cup fresh cilantro

Directions:

1. Coat the slow cooker with cooking spray. Mix the eggs, salt, pepper, plus milk in a bowl.
2. Add garlic powder, cumin, coriander, and sausage and mix well.
3. Pour the mixture into the slow cooker. Set the slow cooker on 'Low' within 4-5 hours or on 'High' for 2-3 hours. Place toppings of your choice and serve.

Nutrition: Calories: 320 Fat: 24.1 g Carb: 5.2 g Protein: 17.9 g

Almond Lemon Blueberry Muffins

Preparation time: 15 minutes

Cooking time: 3 hours

Servings: 3

Ingredients:

- 1 cup almond flour
- 1 large egg
- 3 drops stevia
- ¼ cup fresh blueberries
- ¼ teaspoon lemon zest, grated
- ¼ teaspoon pure lemon extract
- ½ cup heavy whipping cream
- 2 tablespoons butter, melted
- ½ teaspoon baking powder

Directions:

1. Whisk the egg into a bowl. Add the rest of the fixing, and mix.
2. Pour batter into lined or greased muffin molds. Pour up to ¾ of the cup.
3. Pour 6 ounces of water into the slow cooker. Place an aluminum foil at the bottom, and the muffin molds inside.
4. Set the slow cooker on 'High' within 2-3 hours. Let it cool in the cooker for a while.

5. Remove from the cooker. Loosen the edges of the
    muffins. Invert on to a plate and serve.

Nutrition: Calories: 223 Fat: 21g Carb: 5g Protein: 6 g

Healthy Veggie Omelet

Preparation time: 15 minutes

Cooking time: 1 hour & 40 minutes

Servings: 4

Ingredients:

- 6 eggs
- 1 tsp parsley, dried
- 1 tsp garlic powder
- 1 bell pepper, diced
- 1/2 cup onion, sliced
- 1 cup spinach
- 1/2 cup almond milk, unsweetened
- 4 egg whites
- Pepper
- Salt

Directions:

1. Grease the slow cooker from inside using cooking spray.
2. Whisk egg whites, eggs, parsley, garlic powder, almond milk, pepper, and salt in a large bowl.
3. Stir in bell peppers, spinach, and onion. Pour egg batter into the slow cooker.
4. Cook on high within 90 minutes or until egg sets. Cut into the slices and serve.

Nutrition: Calories: 200 Fat: 13.9 g Carb: 5.8 g Protein 13.4 g

Parmesan Zucchini Paprika & Ricotta Frittata

Preparation time: 15 minutes

Cooking time: 6 hours

Servings: 6

Ingredients:

- 2 medium zucchinis, shredded
- 1 teaspoon kosher salt, divided
- 1 tablespoon extra-virgin olive oil
- 12 large eggs
- 3 tablespoons heavy (whipping) cream
- 3 tablespoons finely chopped fresh parsley
- 1 tablespoon fresh thyme
- ½ teaspoon paprika
- ½ teaspoon freshly ground black pepper
- 6 ounces' ricotta cheese
- 12 cherry tomatoes, halved
- ½ cup grated Parmesan cheese

Directions:

1. Toss the shredded zucchini with ½ teaspoon of salt in a colander set in the sink. Let the zucchini sit for a few minutes, then squeeze out the excess liquid with your hands.
2. Grease the slow cooker with olive oil.

3. Beat the eggs, heavy cream, parsley, thyme, paprika, pepper, and the remaining ½ teaspoon of salt in a large bowl.
4. Put the zucchini and stir. Transfer the mixture to the prepared insert.
5. Using a large spoon, dollop the ricotta cheese into the egg mixture, distributing it evenly.
6. Top with the tomatoes and sprinkle the Parmesan cheese over the top. Set to cook within 6 hours on low or 3 hours on high. Serve at room temperature.

Nutrition: Calories: 291 Fat: 22g Carbs: 4g Protein: 18g

Yummy Cauliflower Crust Breakfast Pizza

Preparation time: 15 minutes

Cooking time: 5 hours

Servings: 4

Ingredients:

- 2 large eggs
- 3 cups riced cauliflower
- 1 cup grated Parmesan cheese
- 8 ounces' goat cheese, divided
- ½ teaspoon kosher salt
- 1 tablespoon extra-virgin olive oil
- Grated zest of 1 lemon

Directions:

1. Beat the eggs, cauliflower, Parmesan cheese, 2 ounces of goat cheese, and the salt until well mixed in a large bowl.
2. Grease the slow cooker using the olive oil. Press the cauliflower batter in an even layer around the cooker's bottom and extend slightly up the sides.
3. Stir the remaining 6 ounces of goat cheese and the lemon zest in a small bowl. Dollop spoonsful onto the cauliflower crust, distributing it evenly.
4. Set the lid on the slow cooker, but prop it slightly open with a chopstick or wooden spoon. Cook within

6 hours on low or 3 hours on high, until the edges are slightly browned.

5. When finished, turn off the cooker but let the pizza sit in it 30 minutes before serving. Serve warm.

Nutrition: Calories: 389 Fat: 29g Carbs: 6g Protein: 24g

Arugula Cheese Herb Frittata

Preparation time: 15 minutes

Cooking time: 3 hours & 10 minutes

Servings: 6

Ingredients:

- 8 eggs
- 3/4 cup goat cheese, crumbled
- 1/2 cup onion, sliced
- 1 1/2 cups red peppers, roasted and chopped
- 4 cups baby arugula
- 1 tsp oregano, dried
- 1/3 cup almond milk
- Pepper
- Salt

Directions:

1. Grease the slow cooker using a cooking spray. Whisk eggs, oregano, and almond milk in a mixing bowl.
2. Put pepper and salt. Arrange red peppers, onion, arugula, and cheese into the slow cooker.
3. Pour egg batter into the slow cooker over the vegetables. Cook on low within 3 hours. Serve hot and enjoy.

Nutrition: Calories: 178 Fat: 12.8 g Carb: 6 g Protein: 11.4 g

Cheese Grits

Preparation time : 5 minutes

Cooking time: 5-7 hours

Servings: 4 people

Ingredients:

- 1/2 cup stone-ground grits
- 5-6 cups of water
- 2 tsp salt
- 1/2 cup Cheddar cheese (shredded)
- 6 tbsp butter
- Black pepper (optionally)

Directions:

1. Preheat slow cooker, spray the dish with cooking spray, or cover with butter. In a wide bowl, mix grits and water, add salt. Cook on low temperatures for 5-7 hours; you can leave it overnight.

2. Remove the dish from the slow cooker, cover butter on top. Stir with the whisk to an even consistency and fully melted butter.

3. To serve, sprinkle more cheese on top and black pepper to your taste. Serve warm.

Nutrition: Calories: 173 Fat: 7g Carbohydrates: 4g Protein: 6g

Pineapple Cake with Pecans

Preparation time: 15 minutes

Cooking time: 3-4 hours

Servings: 4 people

Ingredients:

- 2 cups of sugar
- 2 cups plain flour
- 2 eggs
- 4 tbsp vegetable oil
- 1 can pineapple with juice (crushed)
- 1 tsp baking soda
- 1 tsp vanilla extract
- Salt
- For icing:
- 1 cup of sugar
- 1/2 cup butter
- 6 tbsp evaporated milk
- 3tbsp shredded coconut
- 1/2 cup chopped pecans (toasted)

Directions:

1. Preheat your slow cooker to 180-200 degrees. Take a medium bowl and combine all cake ingredients.

2. Mix the dough until evenly combined and then pour into slow cooker dish. Bake for 3 hours on high; check if it is ready with a wooden toothpick.

3. When the cake is ready, make the icing: in a medium saucepan, combine sugar, evaporated milk, butter, and salt. Bring to boil, and then simmer with a lower heat for 10 minutes.

4. Add the coconut to the icing. Put the icing over the hot cake, then sprinkle with nuts. To serve, let the cake cool, then cut it and serve with your favorite drinks.

Nutrition: Calories: 291 Fat: 7g Carbohydrates: 6g Protein: 5g

Potato Casserole for Breakfast

Preparation time: 5 minutes

Cooking time: 4 hours

Servings: 4 people

Ingredients:

- 4 big potatoes
- 5-6 sausages
- 1/2 cup cheddar cheese (shredded)
- 1/2 cup mozzarella cheese
- 5-6 green onions
- 10 chicken eggs
- 1/2 cup milk
- Salt
- Black pepper

Directions:

1. Preheat slow cooker; spray its dish with non-stick cooking spray. Rub the potatoes into small pieces and put them into the dish.

2. Cover the potatoes with rubbed sausages. Add both mozzarella, cheddar cheeses, and green onions. Continue the layers until all space in the dish is full.

3. Mix the wet ingredients (milk, eggs) in a medium bowl. Pour it into the main dish, then put salt and pepper.

Nutrition: Calories: 190 Fat: 10g Carbohydrates: 5g

Protein: 10g

85

Cinnamon Rolls

Preparation time: 15 minutes

Cooking time: 2 hours

Servings: 10-12 pieces

Ingredients:

- 2 cups warm water
- 1 tbsp active yeast (dry)
- 2 tbsp wild honey
- 3 cups plain flour
- 1 tsp salt
- 4 tbsp butter
- 4 tbsp brown sugar
- 1 tsp cinnamon

Directions:

1. In a bowl, mix up water, yeast, and honey. Stir with a mixer and after the dough is homogenous, let it rest for several minutes; mixture will rise.

2. Sift flour and add salt. Mix on low to let the ingredients come together, then increase the mixing speed to medium. Remove dough and allow to rise on a floured table.

3. Roll dough into medium rectangles. You can use a pizza cutter to make the sides even. Spread the

butter over the dough. Sprinkle it with sugar and cinnamon.

4. Roll the dough rectangles into a long log, and then cut it into 10-12 pieces. Cover your slow cooker inside with foil, place the rolls over it and cook on high for 2-3 hours. To serve, use fresh berries or mint leaves.

Nutrition: Calories: 190 Fat: 5g Carbohydrates: 7g Protein: 8g

ìQuinoa Pie

Preparation time: 10 minutes

Cooking time: 4 hours

Servings: 4 people

Ingredients:

- 2 tbsp almond butter
- 2 tbsp maple syrup
- 1 cup vanilla almond milk
- 1 tsp salt
- 1/2 cup quinoa
- 2 chicken eggs
- Cinnamon
- 1/2 cup raisins
- 5 tbsp roasted almonds (chopped)
- 1/2 cup dried apples

Directions:

1. Spray the slow cooker dish with no-stick spray or cover it with foil or parchment paper. In another bowl, mix the almond butter and maple syrup. Melt in a microwave until creamy, about a minute.

2. Add almond milk, salt, and cinnamon, then whisk the mass until it is entirely even. Add the eggs and remaining products, mix well. Preheat your slow cooker to 100-110 degrees.

3. Put the dough into the dish, then place it into the slow cooker. Cook for 3-4 hours on high. To serve, remove the pie out of the dish with a knife. Cool in the refrigerator.

Nutrition: Calories: 174 Fat: 8g Carbohydrates: 20g Protein: 6g

Quinoa Muffins with Peanut Butter

Preparation time: 10 minutes

Cooking time: 4 hours

Servings: 8 muffins

Ingredients:

- 1 cup strawberries
- 1/2 cup almond vanilla milk
- 1 tsp salt
- 5-6 tbsp raw quinoa
- 2 tbsp peanut butter (better natural)
- 3 tbsp honey
- 4 egg whites
- 2 tbsp peanuts (roasted)

Directions:

1. Preheat your slow cooker to 190 degrees. Line the cooking dish bottom with parchment paper; additionally, spray it with cooking spray. Dice the strawberries and place them over the dish.

2. Sprinkle with honey and place the dish into the slow cooker for 10-15 minutes for releasing juices. In another pot, mix up the almond milk and salt. Boil with quinoa until ready.

3. Combine egg whites and almond butter in a separate bowl. Put the quinoa and wait until milk is absorbed.

4. Fill the muffin forms with quinoa mixture; place the strawberries on the top. Bake in the slow cooker on low until quinoa is set for about 4 hours. To serve, cool the muffins and decorate them with whole strawberries.

Nutrition: Calories: 190 Fat: 6g Carbohydrates: 8g Protein: 6g

Veggie Omelets

Preparation time: 5 minutes

Cooking time: 2 hours

Servings: 8 pieces

Ingredients:

- 6 chicken eggs
- 1/2 cup milk
- salt
- garlic powder
- white pepper
- red pepper
- small onion
- garlic clove
- parsley
- 5 small tomatoes

Directions:

1. Grease the slow cooker dish with butter or special cooking spray. In a separate bowl, mix up eggs and milk. Add pepper and garlic.

2. Whisk the mixture well and salt. Add to the mixture broccoli florets, onions, pepper, and garlic. Stir in the eggs.

3. Place the mixture into the slow cooker dish. Cook on high temperatures at 180-200 degrees for 2 hours. Cover with cheese and let it melt. To serve,

cut the omelet into 8 pieces and garnish the plates with parsley and tomatoes.

Nutrition: Calories: 210 Fat: 7g Carbohydrates: 5g Protein: 8g

Apple Pie with Oatmeal

Preparation time: 10 minutes

Cooking time: 4-6 hours

Servings: 4 people

Ingredients:

- 1 cup oats
- 2 large apples
- 2 cups almond milk
- 2 cups warm water
- 2 tsp cinnamon
- Pinch nutmeg
- Salt
- 2 tbsp coconut oil
- 1 tsp vanilla extract
- 2 tbsp flaxseeds
- 2 tbsp maple syrup
- Raisins

Directions:

1. Grease your slow cooker. Rub a couple of spoons of coconut or olive oil. Peel the apples. Core and chop them into medium size pieces.
2. Starting with the apples, add all the ingredients into the slow cooker. Stir and leave to bake for 6 hours on low. When ready, stir the oatmeal well.

3. Serve the oatmeal into small cups. You can also
    garnish it with any berries or toppings you like.

Nutrition: Calories: 159 Fat: 12g Carbohydrates: 9g
Protein: 28g

Vanilla French Toast

Preparation time: 15 minutes

Cooking time: 8 hours/overnight

Servings: 4 people

Ingredients:

- 1 loaf bread (better day-old)
- 2 cups cream
- 2 cups milk, whole
- 8 eggs
- almond extract
- 1 vanilla bean
- 5 tsp sugar
- Cinnamon
- Salt

Directions:

1. Coat the slow cooker dish with the cooking spray. Slice bread into small pieces (1-2 inches). Place them into the dish overlapping each other. In another dish, combine the remaining ingredients until perfectly blended.

2. Pour the wet mixture over the bread to cover it completely. Place the dish into a slow cooker and cook on low at 100-120 degrees for 7-8 hours. To serve, slightly cool and cut the French toast.

Nutrition: Calories: 200 Fat: 6g Carbohydrates: 4g Protein: 8g

Greek Eggs Casserole

Preparation time: 15 minutes

Cooking time: 6 hours

Servings: 4 people

Ingredients:

- 10 chicken eggs
- 1/2 cup milk
- Salt
- 1 tsp black pepper
- 1 tbsp red onion
- 1/2 cup dried tomatoes
- 1 cup champignons
- 2cups spinach
- 1/2 cup feta

Directions:

1. Set your slow cooker to 120-150 degrees. In a separate wide bowl, combine and whisk the eggs. Add salt and pepper. Mix in garlic and red onion. Whisk again.
2. Wash and dice the mushrooms. Put them into the wet mixture. At last, and add dried tomatoes. Pour the mixture into the slow cooker.
3. Top the meal with the feta cheese and cook on low for 5-6 hours. Serve with milk or vegetables.

Nutrition: Calories: 180 Fat: 8g Carbohydrates: 4g Protein: 8g

Treacle Sponge with Honey

Preparation time: 15 minutes

Cooking time: 3 hours

Servings: 4 people

Ingredients:

- 1 cup unsalted butter
- 3 tbsp. honey
- 1 tbsp. white breadcrumbs (fresh)
- 1 cup of sugar
- 1 lemon zest
- 3 large chicken eggs
- 2 cup flour
- 2 tbsp. milk
- Clotted cream (to serve)
- Little brandy splash (optional)

Directions:

1. Grease your slow cooker dish heavily and preheat it. Mix the breadcrumbs with the honey in a medium bowl. Melt butter and beat it with lemon zest and sugar until fluffy and light. Sift in the flour slowly.

2. Add the milk and stir well. Spoon the mixture into the slow cooker dish—Cook for 3 hours on low mode. Serve with honey or clotted cream.

Nutrition: Calories: 200 Fat: 10g Carbohydrates: 20g Protein: 10g

Sticky Pecan Buns with Maple

Preparation time: 15 minutes

Cooking time: 5 hours

Servings: 12 rolls

Ingredients:

- 6 tbsp. milk (nonfat)
- 4 tbsp. maple syrup
- 1/2 tbsp. melted butter
- 1 tsp. vanilla extract
- Salt
- 2 tbsp. yeast
- 2 cup flour (whole wheat)
- Chopped pecans
- Ground cinnamon

Directions:

1. Coat the inside of your slow cooker using a non-stick cooking spray. For the dough, combine milk, vanilla butter, and maple syrup. Mix well.

2. Microwave the mixture until warm and add the yeast. Let sit for 15 minutes. Sift in the flour and mix until the dough is no stickier.

3. For the filling, mix the maple syrup and cinnamon. Roll out the dough and brush it with the maple filling. Roll up, then slice into 10-12 parts. Place the small rolls into the slow cooker.

4. For the caramel sauce, combine milk, butter, and syrup. Pour the sauce into the slow cooker—Cook for 2 hours on high or 5 hours on low. Serve.

Nutrition: Calories: 230 Fat: 5g Carbohydrates: 29g Protein: 42g

Vegetarian Pot Pie

Preparation time: 15 minutes

Cooking time: 9 hours & 15 minutes

Servings: 4 people

Ingredients:

- 6 cups chopped vegetables (peas, potatoes, tomatoes, carrots, Brussels sprouts)
- 1-2 cups diced mushrooms
- 2 onions
- 1/2 cup flour
- 4 cloves garlic
- 2 tbsp. garlic
- Thyme (fresh)
- Cornstarch
- 2 cups chicken broth

Directions:

1. Wash and chop vegetables or by frozen packed. Toss with flour to cover vegetables well.
2. Mix with the broth slowly, when well combined with flour. Preheat the slow cooker and place the vegetables into it.
3. Cook on low for 8-9 hours, or on high for 6-7 hours. Mix up cornstarch with the water and pour into the vegetable mix. Place it back in the slow cooker for 15 minutes. Serve hot with fresh vegetables.

Nutrition: Calories: 267 Fat: 7g Carbohydrates: 29g Protein: 7g

Blueberry Porridge

Preparation time: 5 minutes

Cooking time: 5-6 hours

Servings: 4 people

Ingredients:

- 1 cup jumbo oats
- 4 cups of milk
- 1/2 cup dried fruits
- Brown sugar or honey
- Cinnamon
- Blueberries

Directions:

1. Heat the slow cooker before the start. Put the oats into the slow cooker dish, add some salt.
2. Pour over the milk, then place the dish into the slow cooker and cook on low for 7-8 hours (overnight). Stir the porridge in the morning.
3. For serving, ladle into the serving bowls and decorate with your favorite yogurt or syrup. Add blueberries.

Nutrition: Calories: 210 Fat: 4g Carbohydrates: 5g Protein: 8g

Crock Pot Keto English Muffin

Preparation time: 15 minutes

Cooking time: 2 hours

Servings: 6

Ingredients:

- almond flour3 tablespoons
- coconut flour 1/2 tablespoon
- butter 1 tablespoon
- egg 1 large
- sea salt1 pinch
- baking soda1/2 teaspoons
- salt

Directions:

1. Take a medium-sized skillet, melt the butter. It usually takes 20-30 seconds.
2. Pour coconut and almond flour, egg, salt into the melted butter and stir everything well.
3. Remove skillet from the heat and add baking soda.
4. Coat the slow cooker with cooking spray. Pour the mixture.
5. Put on low for 2 hours. Check the readiness with a fork.
6. Remove the baked muffin from the slow cooker and eat with bacon slices, cheese, or other breakfast staples.

Nutrition: Calories: 188 Carbs: 3g Fat: 17g Protein: 7g

Blueberry Pancake

Preparation time: 15 minutes

Cooking time: 40 minutes

Servings: 8

Ingredients:

- 1½ cups milk
- 2 large eggs
- 1 teaspoon vanilla
- 2 cups all-purpose flour
- 2½ teaspoon baking powder
- 2 tablespoons white sugar
- ¼ cup fresh blueberries

Directions:

1. Toss the eggs, vanilla, and milk together in a small bowl. Stir flour, sugar, and baking powder together in a large bowl until well-mixed.
2. Add the wet fixings to the dry and stir just until mixed.
3. Pour the batter into the slow cooker. Add the blueberries.
4. Set the timer at 40 minutes on low.
5. Check to confirm if the pancake is cooked through by pressing the top. Serve and enjoy with syrup, fruit, or whipped cream.

Nutrition: Calories: 174 Carbs: 30g Protein: 6g Fat: 2g
Cholesterol: 45mg Sodium: 37mg Potassium: 266mg Sugar:
5g